SENSE AND SYNESTHESIA

Previous Books by E T Rook

My Grandmother Was from Wales
Memoir describing the life of Oklahoma pioneer Jane E. Champlin, whose parents immigrated from Wales
(2004)

Senator: 1876-1965 The Life and Career of Senator Elmer Thomas
Historical biography chronicling the background and career of the author's great grandfather, Senator Elmer Thomas (D-OK)
(2015)

Both can be found @ www.etrook.com.

Praise for E T Rook

"*My Grandmother Was from Wales* depicts the heartwarming story of a loving grandmother and close-knit family as can only be seen through the eyes of a grandchild growing up amidst them."

- Millie Craddick, *Oklahoma Heritage Magazine*, Spring/Summer 2005

"What a fantastic author! I recommend you read her books *Senator: 1876-1965* and *My Grandmother Was from Wales*. Betsy is dedicated to her research. She provides all the details so that everyone can be part of her intriguing stories and historical documentation of these unsung heroes."

- Madison Wright, Editor in Chief, Firstediting.com

Sense and Synesthesia

E T Rook

DISCLAIMER

While every precaution has been taken in the preparation of this book, the publisher assumes no responsibility for errors and omissions or for damages resulting from the use of information contained herein.

Cover image: E T Rook, 1991

Edited by First Editing
Layout and cover design by From Manuscript to Book

Copyright © 2024 E T Rook

Rook Publishing

All rights reserved. No part of this publication may be reproduced or transmitted in any form or by any means, electronic or mechanical, including photocopying, recording, or by any information storage and retrieval system, without permission in writing from the author. Reviewers may quote brief passages.

ISBN 979-8-218-67172-3

Printed in the United States of America

Ebook edition available

Contents

Introduction 1
Chapter 1 - Synesthesia: An Overview 5
Chapter 2 - Forms of Synesthesia 13
Chapter 3 - Synesthesia and Drugs 21
Chapter 4 - The Brain and Theories of Synesthesia 27
Chapter 5 - Synesthesia and Everyday Life 35
Chapter 6 - My Synesthesia 47
Chapter 7 - Experiments in Synesthesia 69
Chapter 8 - Personal Accounts of Synesthesia 77
Acknowledgements 81
Bibliography 83
References 85
Index 92

List of Illustrations

Figure 1	Mysid, 20 August 2007. Synesthesia Colored Numbers	9
Figure 2	Galton, 1881. Number Form.	9
Figure 3	Kluver, 1926. Form Constants.	20
Figure 4	MacLean, 1990. Triune Brain.	28
Figure 5	Rook, W.E. 2024. Mango.	36
Figure 6	Rook, E.T. 2022. Sweden and Thankfulness.	37
Figure 7	Rook, W.E., 2023. Young Man Turning into a Chair.	39
Figure 8	Retgien, 2007. Alphabet Colors and Spatial Forms.	44
Figure 9	Rook, E.T. 2022. The Numbers Spelled Out.	48
Figure 10	Rook, E.T. 2022. The Numbers, Digits.	48
Figure 11	Rook, E.T. 2022. The Days of the Week (Text)	49
Figure 12	Rook, E.T. 2022. The Days of the Week (Colors).	49
Figure 13	Rook, E.T. 2022. The Months of the Year (Text)	50
Figure 14	Rook, E.T. 2022. The Months of the Year (Colors)	50
Figure 15	Rook, E.T. 2022. Umbrella.	52
Figure 16	Rook, E.T. 2022. Chloroform.	53
Figure 17	Rook, E.T. 2022. Spinning.	53
Figure 18	Rook, E.T. 2022. Break.	55
Figure 19	Rook, E.T. 2022. Brake.	55
Figure 20	Rook, E.T.2022. The Alphabet (Text).	61
Figure 21	Rook, E.T. 2022. The Alphabet (Colors).	61
Figure 22	Mondrian, 1918, and 1942-1944. Composition with Grey Lines and Victory Boogie Woogie	74

Dedicated to Bonnie

Introduction

Back in 1980, I was about to graduate Oklahoma State University and I was lucky enough to be in Boulder, Colorado, visiting my good family friend Bonnie Crumpacker, her husband Wilson, and family during a March spring school break. I didn't know Bonnie or Wilson very well, but I was so glad when they both welcomed me into their fold, and I spent many a happy hour talking and reminiscing with them both as Wilson was my maternal grandfather's sister's husband's cousin!! Which, according to a Google search, is my third cousin once removed. Their family used to visit quite often in Oklahoma when I was a child, but although we knew one another, we never were close. I had a large family, and as the community was small and fairly tight-knit we talked a lot about the "the good old days."

One of these times, as I was spending quite an informative and relaxing day with Bonnie, I happened to mention that I remembered dates and certain names, etc. by associating them with different colors. Each number and each letter had a specific color hue, and no matter what I did, this "color-coded memory" which I called it, did not go away. It was emblazoned in my consciousness for all time.

She thought that was just absolutely the best thing that anyone had ever told her, and immediately started asking me all sorts of questions about it, most of which I couldn't answer, at least not as fully as I would have liked. She asked how this process got started, if I could control it, if it was something that I had always had. I told her I could not remember how it started, only that I first became aware of it when I was in kindergarten, I could not control it, that it was totally spontaneous and unplanned. At that point she told me about a book she had read about young women from some far away place or islands; I can't remember the title of the book, unfortunately, but somehow she believed these islander women had visions, or sensations, which she believed were similar to my sensations. It could have been even the Maoris of New Zealand, and upon researching, the Maori are known to have a higher prevalence of this trait. Neither one of us knew at the time that the trait that I had would be called synesthesia, which, in general terms, we know now is when one sense is triggered by another sense, and about 4% of the population is known to have. We talked some more about it, and shared a few laughs on the incredulousness of the entire situation, and pretty much I thought no more about it for a long, long time. Bonnie suggested, at some point, that I should write a book about my unique relationship with colors. Although touched by her seemingly admiring perspective on my ability, I was not fully able to appreciate the scope and gravity of her book idea. But I did feel validated and I must admit I wanted to think that I might have some special talent that was truly remarkable which was quite uncommon. So I tucked away my 'special talent' for many years and only brought it up to people I trusted, and as not anyone in my family had ever mentioned they had it, I did not bring it up. Actually I believe I did tell my family at some point; but if I ever did try and explain the reason why I remembered them, the "color-coded memory" did not impress them as it had my friend Bonnie.

Fast forward to the early 21st century. I am at my gym, I'm married, with two young children, and I'm working out. I glance up to a magazine rack and I see an article in *Newsweek* titled "Synesthesia*:* The Wonderful World of Color," or something similar. I do a double take, peer at the word with as much scientific memory as I can muster, and quickly realize in an instant that I am not alone. I file the experience away for later, but still, I do not pursue it.

I will get to that someday, I said, and that someday is now. Still, it took another almost 20 years after the *Newsweek* article to take on this book. After not being studied much for decades throughout the early 20th century, the tide turned in the 1980s, about the time I told Bonnie about mine. Synesthesia is quite the topic now.

I only wish Bonnie were here to see I did write that book. Thank you, dear friend.

CHAPTER 1

Synesthesia: An Overview

Synesthesia means the "joined sensation" and, according to Richard Cytowic in *Wednesday Is Indigo Blue* (2011), this means a combination, or the overlap of more than one sense, such as sight, sound, touch, smell, or taste (1). For example, a person may hear a word, such as "oral" and see a color, or several colors. For example, the letters "o," "r," "a," and "l" may all induce a specific color in the synesthete's mind.

One out of every four people may have some form of synesthesia, but there have been many studies done on this, and they have all resulted in varying percentages within the population.

The most common form, grapheme color, is found in about one percent of the population. One study by the University of Glasgow found that about four percent of the general population have it, with nine varying forms of synesthesia. At one time, it was thought that females were more likely to have the trait, but recent studies have found it is equal between men and women (Day, 2024).

In *Synesthesia* (2018), Cytowic said there is a fifty percent chance of having another form if a person has one type already. Often, the synesthesia flows in one direction, meaning that if you hear sounds and have a color concurrent, it will flow only in that direction, but there are some persons in which the flow is bidirectional (3).

In her book, *Synesthesia: The Fascinating World of Blended Senses* (2013), Lindsay Leatherdale contends that sixty-two percent of the population with synesthesia have the grapheme color type, and there are sixty different varieties of synesthesia (11). Although synesthesia is hard to diagnose, one of the main ways the trait can be discovered is in the synesthesia questionnaire, which may have several strategically placed questions designed to extricate the responses from potential synesthesia candidates whether they have the trait (42).

Many artists are not synesthetic, but they do use the form in their work, meaning that they do not subconsciously and automatically have these types of images with sounds of visual stimulation, but they apply metaphors, comparing two senses in their artistic and intellectual expression (Cytowic 2018, 15-16).

In the anthology, *Synaesthesia: Classic and Contemporary Readings* (1997), Cytowic states that synesthesia is an elementary trait in the brain; it is not elaborate and is emotional and experiential. He also says most people are born with the trait.

It is just that some, due to an inherited physical trait, are more conscious of the experiences within the brain, as explained later in this book. Cytowic also found, at one time, a decreased cortical metabolism during the experience, but the more recent studies indicate more cortical involvement than previously thought, according to Sean Day, PhD, and President of IASAS (International Association of Synesthetes, Artists, and Scientists) (Day, 2024). In Cytowic's definition, synesthesia is a conscious awareness of the holistic process of perception that is prematurely displayed (38).

Most people who have synesthesia are not even aware of the trait. They can also assume everyone has the trait, and it is nothing unusual. In this author's case, I was not aware that most people did not associate colors with the days of the week until I was in my mid-twenties. I was fortunate that the person I talked with about my "associations" was highly complimentary, and thought it a talent. Some with synesthesia report negative consequences, such as sensory overload or problems with math, such as this author, but most who have it say synesthesia impacts their life in a positive way, such as being able to be more creative in art, music, literature, and being able to memorize information or names and places. Some say their synesthesia helps them to learn languages, and history, with dates. Most who have it also say they are glad they have it, and life without it would be less interesting.

Synesthesia is not included in the *Diagnostic and Statistical Manual of Mental Disorders* (DSM-V), and is not thought to impair mental function in any way. While most with synesthesia seem to appreciate their different way of perceiving their senses, there is a type of synesthesia, misophonia, which can result in certain sounds causing strong, unbearable feelings. For example, the sound of a barking dog could cause a person with misophonia to experience strong feelings of disgust or sadness. Fortunately, this is quite rare.

There are several factors which determine whether a person has the neurological trait of synesthesia. According to Cytowic's article "Phenomenology and Neuropsychology" (1997):

1) The responses themselves are consistent and do not vary over time.

2) They are simple and laden with affect, meaning they are related to emotion and the expression of emotion.

3) Synesthesia is highly memorable, totally involuntary, and an automatic response which is not fore planned or given to any grandiose brain function by the synesthete (24-25).

In *Wednesdays Are Indigo Blue*, Richard Cytowic says that number forms, or grapheme color synesthesia that involves only numbers, can be spatially extended as in localizers, or non-spatially extended, as in non-localizers. This is when a synesthete sees numbers, such as 1-10, in their mind's eye, or hanging somewhere in the air. The mind's eye way is called a localization, and the hanging in the air is called spatially extended (Cytowic, 2011, 72).

SYNESTHESIA
0123456789

Figure 1 Mysid, 20 August 2007. Synesthesia Colored Numbers.

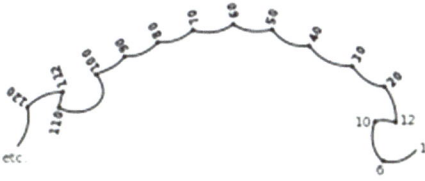

Figure 2 Galton, 1881. Number Form.

The first known case of synesthesia was in 1812. In the mid-20th century, synesthesia was not studied because it was thought that if science could not explain it, then it could not be studied. After the 1950s, the paradigm began to shift, and synesthesia was thought to explain how abstract thinking develops, along with creativity (Cytowic 2018, 20-28).

Cretien van Campen points out in his book, *The Hidden Sense*, that most testing for determining whether a person has synesthesia is done through a consistency test. However, the test revealed discrepancies when the colors, although consistent, could not be measured due to multiple variations (124). Van Campen says the question is not whether a person is a synesthete, but how much of a synesthete you are, because almost everyone has some measure of synesthesia; it is just how much consciousness of sensory processes a person has that is the determining factor (127).

In *Psychology Today*, Laura Moss says that many synesthetes say having it helps with memory, as words such as names and dates are associated with colors. In 2004, University of California students took a Torrance Test of Creative Thinking and synesthetes scored twice as high as non-synesthetes in each category.

Painter Vincent Van Gogh, actress Marilyn Monroe, singer-songwriter Mary J. Blige, and record producer Pharrell Williams are all synesthetes. Williams told *Psychology Today* he "associates music with colors and can't imagine making music without it" (Moss).

In *Synesthesia: Classic and Contemporary Readings,* in the chapter titled "Phenomenology and Neuropsychology: A Review of Current Knowledge" by Baron-Cohen and John E.Harrison, the ratio for synesthetes is said to be 3:1 female to male in the US and 8:1 female to male in the UK (Cytowic 1997, 19).

Furthermore, the study of synesthesia is likely to cause concerns about the ethics of brain study, as synesthesia is largely an inheritable trait (115).

CHAPTER 2

Forms of Synesthesia

In Lyndsay Leatherdale's book *Synesthesia: The Fascinating World of Blended Senses,* the following list provides a breakdown of various kinds of synesthesia and their corresponding percentages of the population:

- 62.5% grapheme color—numbers
- 21.9% have sound—vision
- 19.3% music—flavors
- 14.72% sounds—color
- 8.92% personalities—color
- 8.7% mirror—touch (other people's sensations)
- 6.66% phonemes—color
- 6.23% flavors—color
- 5.91% smells—touch
- 5.2% pain—color

These numbers are of all synesthetes, and not of the entire population.

The second most common form of synesthesia is colored hearing, or chromesthesia, where a person will hear sounds, sometimes musical notes, and see different colors displayed in their mind's eye, or even sometimes suspended in the air outside of their body (9).

These two different ways of seeing the colors are called projective and associative, and have been discussed in Chapter One as localizers and non-localizers. Associative or localized is when a person sees the color or resulting perception in the mind's eye, and projective, or non-localized, is when a person sees the response projected in front of them, as if the colors were "hanging in the air." The other terms of description are "localizers" and "non-localizers" or "spatially extended."

The other more common forms of synesthesia include touch synesthesia or mirror-touch synesthesia, when a person sees someone being touched and responds by feeling the same touch on their body; grapheme personification, when numbers are given different personalities; and misophonia, when experiencing different emotions when triggered by sounds; lexical-gustatory synesthesia, when a person tastes flavors within certain words or letters or sees corresponding shapes; and spatial-sequence, when a person sees the corresponding colors to words or months of the year in the space near to, but outside of, their body. A rarer form of synesthesia involves the sense of smell, when a person smells various types of smells when presented with words (Wikipedia, "Synesthesia").

In *Wednesdays Are Indigo Blue* (2011), Cytowic states that taste and smell senses are organized differently in the brain from vision and hearing, and that Michael Watson, the main subject of Cytowic's book *The Man Who Tasted Shapes*, who had flavor-touch synesthesia, had polymodal synesthesia. Michael, when triggered by tastes or smells, would see different colored shapes and patterns, and would also feel tactile sensations depending on the type of taste or odor (133).

In *Synesthesia* (2018), Cytowic says the term 'flavor' can mean both taste and smell, and triggers shapes, colors, and visceral patterns with different forms. This is illustrated again by Cytowic's patient Watson, who, when tasting certain flavors, felt tactile sensations, forms, and patterns which could be felt and seen (107). The more common a word, the stronger the flavor (127). As for this author's synesthesia with sight and taste, there is a link between letters and tastes, but not with phonemes. For instance, the word "crying" would be a sensation of wetness, and the color yellowish-white. But the "cry" as in cryosurgery, would not have the same concurrent, or simultaneous sensory perception, as "crying." It would be associated with white, but more with cleanliness or smoothness and not wetness.

Cytowic further expounds that forty percent of synesthetes see with their ears (129). Photisms appear when triggered by sounds, shapes, phonemes, and musical notes. Responses are more than just colors; there is often a spatial mapping of patterns and shapes. These can be in response to pitch, key, timbre, volume, and melody. The French composer Olivier Eugene Prosper Charles Messiaen (1908-1992), who was also an ornithologist and organist, saw complex color patterns in response to different musical notes. His synesthesia was bidirectional in that he saw colors when he heard musical notes, and he translated landscapes into musical notes (143).

In the case of grapheme synesthesia, some letters have stronger colors than others and, predominantly, vowels reflect a stronger color than consonants, but that is not always the case. Sometimes, the first letter of the word dictates what the main color of the word is, but that is not a hard and fast rule, either. Moreover, a word can sound the same, but has a totally different meaning. In this case, it is the spelling of the word and not the meaning that shapes what color that word may be. For example, the word "rain" and "rein" sound the same, but the two words have different meanings. Depending on what colors the letters "r," "a," "i," "e," and "n" are, the two words could have different corresponding colors. Grapheme color synesthetes, as a group, tend to see some vowels with many of the same colors, for instance "o" is often either black or white, "a" is red, and "s" tends to be yellow. But as no two synesthetes can agree on most colors, this is only a generalization, and the varying responses cannot be scientifically pinpointed, which is an interesting element of the trait (Cytowic, 66-67). The example in Chapter Four of the word "break" and "brake" explains this in grapheme color synesthesia, in which the sound of the word does not influence the corresponding color, but the differing letters do produce a different color.

In *Wednesdays Are Indigo Blue*, the most common grapheme color form is with days of the week and the months of the year. Graphemes are more common than phonemes for synesthetic response, and the first letter of a word can sometimes seem to "shade" the rest of the word, depending on the synesthete's unique brain. For others, "apple" is red, because "a" is always red, and the rest of the letters in the word "apple" do not seem to exert as much of an effect on the word's color. As vowels tend to be more strongly colored than consonants, they usually influence almost any word, whether at the beginning or not, such as the word "cart," where "a" is red, thus, the word "cart" has a red tinge to it (68).

An essay by Lawrence E. Marks, "On Colored Hearing Synesthesia: Cross-Modal Translations of Sensory Dimensions" (1997) in *Synesthesia: Classic and Contemporary Readings*, provides general agreement between pitch and brightness in colored hearing, and between colors and vowels. It is thought that even certain sounds evoke colors from these vowels (57). In colored hearing, pitch does determine the lightness or darkness of photisms and it appears that frequency of association and not strength determine the data of the findings. Higher-pitched sounds are smaller; lower pitched are larger. There seems to be a connection between the way synesthetes see visions of color and the way sounds are colored as well, in that the components of brightness and size are triggered by both auditory and visual sensations (71). In 1933, neuroscientist Newman discovered that the dimensions of brightness and loudness are the same for both kinds of synesthesia, and even for non-synesthetes. From person to person, the responses may vary, but they are always consistent over time, as in grapheme color synesthesia (75).

Another type of sensory response that is related to synesthesia, but is not actually synesthesia, is an automated sensory meridian response. This is characterized by sounds such as music, or even the crinkling of paper, which incites a physical response on the skin, such as hairs tingling. While synesthesia is triggered by sense and elicits a sensory concurrent, auditory sounds trigger ASMR, and elicit a physical response (Wikipedia, "Autonomous Sensory Meridian Response").

Synesthesia (2018) lists five individual group couplings of synesthesia. The first is colored sequences; then colored music;

affective perceptions such as emotion, touch, taste, or smell; nonvisual couplings which can include sound to smell and vision to smell, such as smell, sound and taste; and spatial sequences (Cytowic, 60).

Grapheme personification synesthesia, where emotions are involved in giving certain numbers personalities, involves the projection of feelings onto others, clairvoyance, and auras (161). Everyone, whether synesthetic or not, can relate to the basic pattern form constants, which Kluver discovered as discussed earlier (164). The constants are entwined with meaning and are a part of a person's basic emotional makeup. This goes along with synesthetes being more intuitive and emotionally intelligent than non-synesthetes.

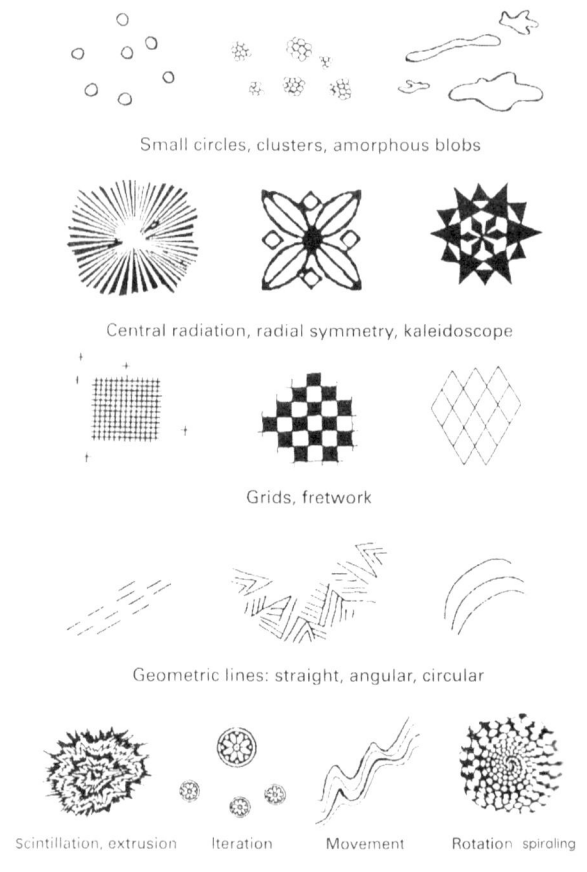

Figure 3   Kluver, 1926. Form Constants.

CHAPTER 3

Synesthesia and Drugs

There are roughly thirty-seven genes which play a factor in synesthesia, but there is no one gene for synesthesia. Studies have found that most persons are born with the mechanism, but most lose the ability to recall the responses as they mature, due to the brain's natural ability to prune the neural fibers involved as the person grows (Price 2018).

A University of Brighton study found learning was a stimulus to the response of synesthesia, as people are not born with synesthetic associations with graphemes. Synesthesia can emerge *de novo*, meaning without any prior family history (Day, 2024). Again, the studies revealed that because synesthesia is perceived as extremely individualized and quite spontaneous, those with it have an instant connection to creating art, music, and literature. (Cohut 2018).

In contrast to his book, *Wednesdays Are Indigo Blue*, in *The Man Who Tasted Shapes* (2003), Cytowic provides more criteria for the synesthesia diagnosis. The following are the underlying hallmarks of synesthesia: it is involuntary, elicited, memorable, durable, and emotional. According to Sean Day, only about 10-15% of persons with visual synesthesia are projectors (Day, 2024).

Many of these, in turn, are polymodal; that is, they have more than one kind of synesthesia. American painter Jane Bowerman has color visions when triggered by shape, movement, or emotion; French composer Olivier Messiaen had bi-directional synesthesia, and saw colors when he heard music, and he would write music when he saw colors. (Cytowic, 2011,94). Other artists, such as Georgia O'Keefe, did not have synesthesia, but applied intellect to their work, in that the responses they painted were not actual responses but were well-thought-out artistic expressions where thought was employed and not an innate, spontaneous, subconscious expression.

In *The Man Who Tasted Shapes*, Cytowic says synesthesia is like altered states of consciousness, but there are differences in these states depending on the pathology behind them. Photographic memory, LSD and release hallucinations, temporal lobe epilepsy, and sensory deprivation all cause a blocking of the sensation to the limbic system, or an increase in activity in the limbic system (126).

The auditory/visual synesthete Michael Watson had spatially extended synesthesia, and was what is called a "localizer" because his sensations were localized to his physical body. Cytowic found certain drugs either suppressed or heightened the sensations in his brain. For instance, amyl nitrite and alcohol increased synesthesia sensations and decreased cortical activity, but amphetamines had the opposite effect by decreasing synesthesia, and heightening the higher cortical brain function. Indeed, during synesthetic episodes, Cytowic found through PET scans that the blood flow in Watson's brain cortex was markedly less than the lowest baseline reading, leading Cytowic to believe that synesthesia occurred in the brain's limbic area, not in the cortex (150). Cytowic emphasized how important the limbic system is to the functioning of the brain and its influence on our behavior. It has a greater impact on the cortex than the cortex on the limbic system. Thus, our emotions influence human behavior more than we know. Humans are guided by emotions and irrationality, not by reason and rationality. It is exactly this emotional element that makes synesthesia so essential, so human (163).

In van Campen's book, *The Hidden Sense: Synesthesia in Art and Science*, he outlines the difference between drug induced and true synesthesia. Drug induced synesthesia is only temporary, disruptive, perceptions constantly change, and it requires drugs, whereas developmental/true synesthesia is constant, the perceptions are consistent, and it usually only enhances a person's perspective (113).

Other methods of inducing synesthesia are with drugs, such as LSD, and meditation. Many meditators experience sound, taste, and touch with emotion, thoughts, and images. In those with temporal lobe epilepsy, seizures cause pain and vision and hearing responses (Cytowic 2003, 135).

In *Synesthesia,* Cytowic comments that although there are many ways synesthesia can be induced through drugs, meditation, brain damage, or epilepsy, there are more differences between acquired synesthesia and developmental synesthesia. Drugs affect perception, and do not induce photisms in regular synesthesia (Cytowic 2018, 211). A person who is more likely to develop synesthesia would be intuitive, and certain outside agents can modify developmental synesthesia, such as alcohol, caffeine, and other drugs. With LSD, the photisms vanish, and the concurrents are emotional. The colors induced by drugs are mainly primary colors, whereas with regular synesthesia, they are many hued and quite varied (212).

In *Synesthesia: Classic and Contemporary Readings* (1997), Edmund M.R.Critchley states in his essay "Synesthesia: Possible Mechanisms" that there are three possible mechanisms for the transmission of synesthetic responses. The first is by crosstalk, or the flow of external input through the sensory channels, leading to the synesthetic perception; the second is release phenomena such as hallucinations and delusions; and the last is the connectivity between the emotions and the actual language and memory (260).

CHAPTER 4

The Brain and Theories of Synesthesia

In *The Man Who Tasted Shapes* (2003), Cytowic states that synesthesia forms in the limbic brain system, and not the cerebral cortex, where most neurologists had thought the trait began. The limbic system guides the emotional responses to stimuli, and the cortex is more responsible for higher functions, such as computing incoming information. However, outdated testing methods were used, and subsequent studies have found there is activity in the cortex with synesthesia. The model of the brain in the book shows three parts of the brain: a lower-level primary part for the sight, sound, and touch sense, where damage caused a total loss of function; a paleomammalian part for the next higher level, with distortion induced by damage; and a neo mammalian for the highest, which was involved in only the highest level of associations (20).

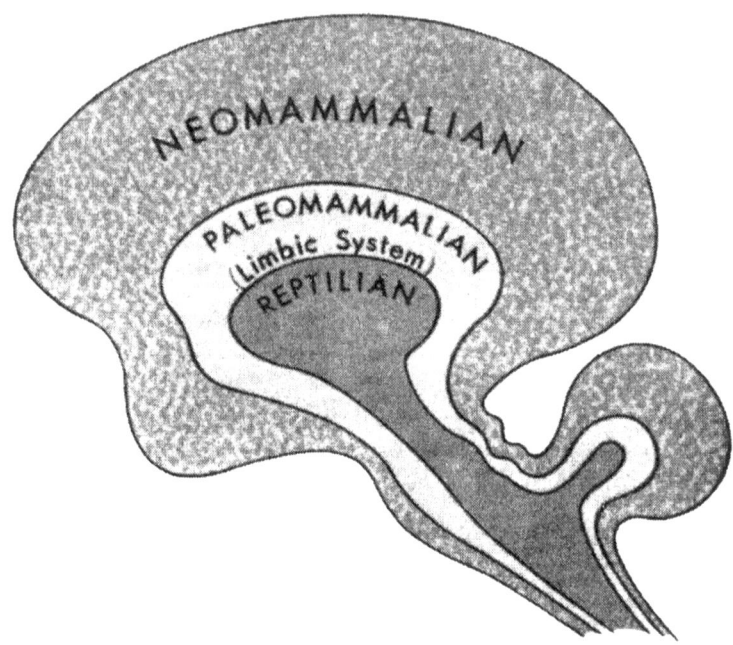

Figure 4   MacLean, 1990. Triune Brain.

In *Synesthesia: Classic and Contemporary Readings*, Frith and Paulescu (1997) state that there are few studies that demonstrate the basis of the beginnings of synesthesia in the brain. Richard Cytowic and neurologist Frank Wood found there is a marked decrease in blood flow within the neocortex during the synesthetic experience with the use of the positron emission tomography (PET) brain scan. This brain area was active in the visual 1 and visual 2 areas. However, in a study by Zeki and Frackoviack, no activity showed that the brain was conscious of precepts without contribution from a primary area

(125). Results of some PET scan studies on women with word/color synesthesia by Frith and Paulescu concluded the brain registered activation in areas of language, and in synesthetes there was more activation within the area of the middle frontal gyrus, the insula on the right, and the posterior inferior temporal (PIT), on the left (125).

In 1995, Frith and Paulescu conducted a study with six synesthetic women with matched controls. The study found abnormal activation in the cortical areas, thus paving the way to a conclusion that some breakdowns of neuronal processes are responsible for synesthesia, and not information processing (128).

Color/word sensation can be evoked by not just a primary visual brain area, but also by other high-level brain areas such as the cortex, and these are where the boundaries for two different senses are likely to overlap (143). There is a feed forward mechanism between language and visual areas, meaning that when an inducer is presented to a synesthete, the inducer, such as a word or a musical note, can induce a color or smell, depending on the kind of synesthete within the person's consciousness.

Furthermore, in Harrison and Baron-Cohen's anthology, *Synesthesia: Classic and Contemporary Readings* (1977), Grossenbacher writes in his essay "Perception and Sensory Information in Synesthetic Experience," that "color was found to be the most dominant concurrent, and trumped the visual precepts such as size and shape. Both normal and synesthetic processing have common neuroanatomical foundations (155). Crosstalk between the neural pathways from a low to a high hierarchy is what forms synesthetic responses in the brain. The goal of the researcher is to find at which level the crosstalk occurs between these two brain wirings and at what level the inducer—the stimuli—influences the concurrent, sensory experience. If both the inducer and the concurrent areas are near each other, there is more chance of crosstalk between these two areas (161). In the feedback model of synesthetic experience, low to high connectivity is stressed.

After various research and more studies, Cytowic noted in *The Man Who Tasted Shapes* (2003) that synesthesia does not occur at the highest nor the lowest level of brain function, but somewhere in the middle (91). He set out to pinpoint exactly where this interaction between stimulus and response took place. He came up with a questionnaire for synesthesia, which had five diagnostic criteria. It is like seeing only without the eyes, in which there is a unity of the senses. It is otherworldly (76).

In *Synesthesia: Classic and Contemporary Readings*, eight theories of how synesthesia develops in the brain are mapped out. The first theory is the neural cognitive connection theory, studied by Dehay, Kennedy, and Bullier, where both auditory and visual brain area pathways are transitory (Baron-Cohen and Harrison 2003, 110). The neurologists Luekowicz and Turkowicz both believed, based upon their studies of infants, that all infants retained these short-lived paths, but they were pruned as the brain matures through childhood into adulthood.

In the sensory leakage theory, information from the auditory area may leak into the visual area of the brain. In Richard Cytowic's theory, information is disconnected from the auditory or visual areas and the limbic system takes over, where the photisms rise to the conscious level within the brain (112). With the learned association theory, information learned in early childhood, such as days of the week or the alphabet, is associated with colors and this sticks in the memory (114). With the genetic theory of synesthesia, the disease is inherited and there may be an opening for these pathways if the neural fibers are not pruned in infancy (115). The environmental maturation theory stresses the direct link between auditory and visual pathways and stresses that early visual information may be a catalyst for synesthesia (116). In the cross-modal theory, studies found that auditory and visual information did interact, and that these interactions were the same for both synesthetes and non-synesthetes alike. And lastly, with the modularity theory, both auditory and visual factors are functionally discreet in non-synesthetes; whereas, in synesthetes, a breakdown in modularity occurs (117).

In the same book, *Synesthesia: Classic and Contemporary Readings*, Daphne Maurer's essay "Neonatal Synesthesia: Implications for the Processing of Faces and Speech" suggests that infants show some cross-modal transfer in early infancy, but most forms of the cross-modal transfer between senses do not emerge till the end of the first year (1997, 225). Young babies less than two months old preferred an optimal level of stimulation, and gave attention to a familiar energy pattern of an object, regardless of the sense of modality.

Likewise, Daphne Maurer argues in this essay that when the cortex is not functioning well, cross-modal confusion can occur, and an infant's brain does experience much sensory confusion (Maurer, 229). As the infant matures, the cortex develops, and the baby can make distinctions between whether he/she is seeing, feeling, or tasting an object. In summary, early infancy babies are synesthetic, but these immature responses decrease as the baby matures, with an increase in sensory cross-modal transfer as the baby reaches its first birthday (236).

As mentioned, synesthesia is associated with math dyscalculia, directional confusion, and a bad sense of direction. Additionally, the trait may also be the flip side of autism, as neural crosstalk is reduced in autism, but increased in synesthesia (Cytowic, 243). Findings indicate about 20% of those on the autistic spectrum have at least one type of synesthesia (Day, 2024). Surely, further study will bear some more cogent and important findings on the subject.

CHAPTER 5

Synesthesia and Everyday Life

There are quite a few literary projects which underscore the importance of synesthesia in not only the lives of those who have the trait but also the lives of those around them. In *A Mango-Shaped Space* (2005) by Wendy Mass, a young girl named Mia learns to appreciate her synesthesia. Though at first she does not understand it at all, she comes to realize, with the help of her family and others in her community, that it is a special gift and can be used in good ways. Mia has at least two kinds of synesthesia; one, she has grapheme color, where letters and numbers have colors, and two, she has colored hearing, where sounds elicit different colors. Her cat, Mango, the subject and title of the book, has a synesthetic color name, because Mia sees an orange mango color when she thinks of her cat, and believes the soul of her late grandfather is within Mango as well. As Mia traverses her eighth grade world, her best friend, meeting boys, professionals helping her, her siblings, and her relationship with her beloved grandfather and her cat, she questions her talent and slowly discovers her power really is special. She also realizes, albeit in her own time, that her gift can help her. Other people will also appreciate it as well.

Books such as *A Mango-Shaped Space* are important as they give people an understanding, from a fictional perspective, of the importance of synesthesia and how it can affect the lives of so many with the trait. When people can read about others and relate to their life events on a personal level, the possibilities are opened not only for broad comprehension of the synesthesia components but also for compassion, and knowledge that they, too, are not alone, and may potentially help others one day.

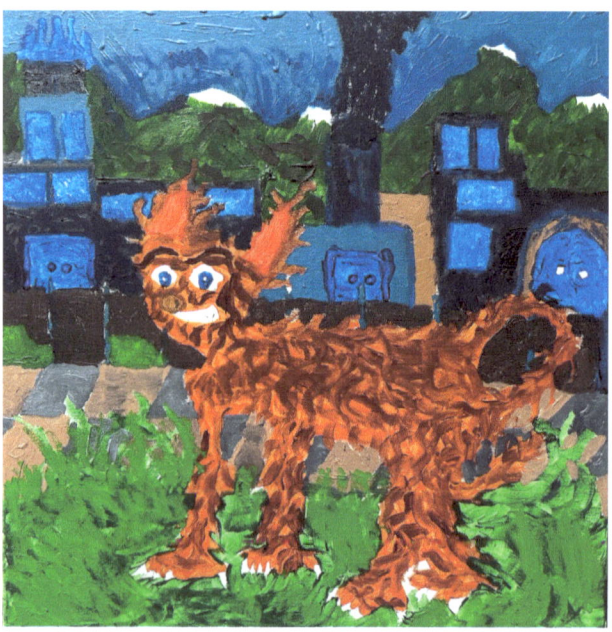

Figure 5   Rook, W.E. 2024. Mango.

In *Synesthesia: Classic and Contemporary Readings,* Alison Motluck's essay, "Two Synesthetes Talking Color" (1997), demonstrates that not everyone with the trait is aware they have it. Ms. Motluck had the pleasure of conversing with British painter Elizabeth Stewart Jones in 1995 who spoke of words being their own color, although the letters of the words also had their individual colors, as is common with synesthetes. Stewart Jones' synesthesia was quite different because of the intricacies of the textures and colors woven into the words and the resulting sensory responses (274). For instance, the word "Sweden" was yellow with a touch of brown and green, and "thankfulness" was red with dark purple. Fig. 6 illustrates the author's colors for "Sweden" and "thankfulness."

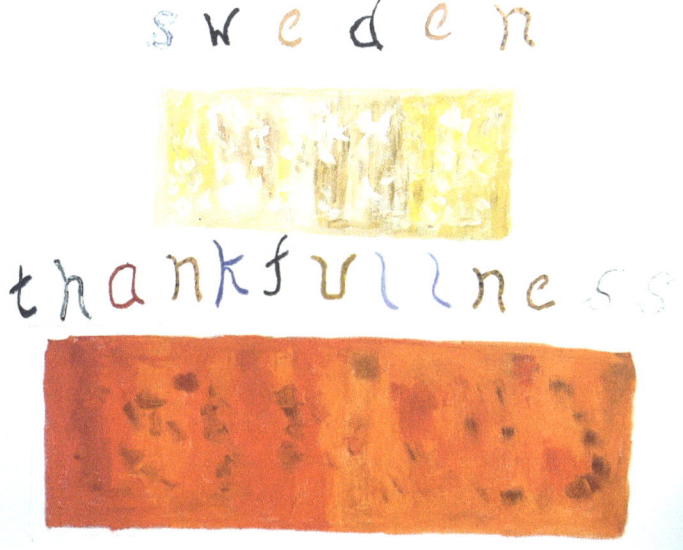

Figure 6   Rook, E.T. 2022. Sweden and Thankfulness.

Numbers also were different in the written and digital form. With the discovery that others also had this ability of making sensory connections between two extremely disparate senses, Ms. Motluck realized that although the processes may be similar, they are not the same for everyone in synesthesia, as different types of synesthetes respond differently to various stimuli.

In *The Particular Sadness of Lemon Cake* by Aimee Bender, a young girl realizes she can experience emotions within the food she tastes, and while this is not a form of synesthesia per se, it is like synesthesia, in that upon the stimulation of one sense (taste), the person feels another concurrent sense (emotion). Rose is raised in a family where emotions are repressed, and feelings are not discussed, and this is her way of bringing them to the surface, although she does not discover her own findings on the food until she is nine years old, and does not express this "magical" way of relating to the world until she is much older. The other family members, her father, who is also repressed, much like Rose, and her mother, who Rose finds to be sad and neglected by her father in her emotional epiphanies, all seem to have the same sort of "different" way of relating to their emotions. But it is her brother that has the darkest and strangest quality of turning himself into inanimate objects, and it makes a sad statement that unexpressed feelings and emotions can take a toll on those that do not recognize them or experience them. While these powers are not scientifically part of synesthesia, it is perhaps wise to take the lessons of this book and apply them to our own lives, and try to discover and excavate emotions, because after all, that is part of what synesthesia is. There is a whole world in the subconscious which is hidden, and colors, words, emotions, and music, amongst others, can help realize this covert world.

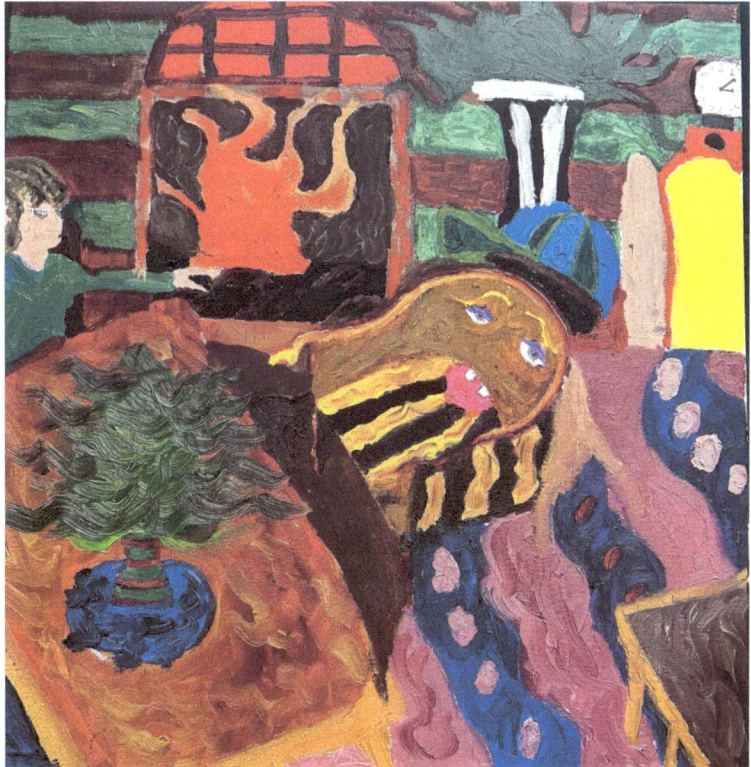

Figure 7   Rook, W.E., 2023. Young Man Turning into a Chair.

In *Blue Cats and Chartreuse Kittens* by Patricia Lynne Duffy, the author recounts the time when she and her dad made word designs and different colors for the words (9). There is a genetic basis for synesthesia, and no two people's synesthetic colors are alike. More recent research has found that the genes related to synesthesia are multisomal, meaning they are found on many different chromosomes, and are not on the X chromosome, refuting findings of the past, according to Sean Day (Day, 2024). There are studies that have shown these genes affect brain maturation, link the cellular connections between sensory modes, and produce abnormal firing between cells (28). Even though the forms may be the same, there are still many variations within the forms, as the same letters in two different languages can have a different color, or texture, or both. Duffy also explains how people can have a different approach to synesthesia; some regard it as an oddity, others as a sensibility, and still others as a form of transcendence (41). The author describes a meeting with Carol Steen, synesthete and visual and sculptural artist, who says her colors are different from the author's. The purpose of Ms. Sheen's artistry is to show the unseen connectedness between different things. Some synesthetes also see colors with pain, as found in studies by neuroscientist Peter Grossenbacher (54).

Those with grapheme color synesthesia often have a certain way of "seeing" their colors in their head, which is only pertinent to certain individuals. Other individuals will see their colors differently in their head, or some, not at all. This is called a number line, discussed earlier as spatially extended number forms, and is very specific, according to the exact color and pattern of organization of the person's idiosyncratic way of perceiving their color pattern. Those synesthetes who can remember every word on a page are seen to have a photographic memory; others, such as Professor Chester from Cornell University, can recall mathematical problems according to their colors, and even formulate the solutions to the problems using their colors (73). Often, no two persons with grapheme color synesthesia have the same colors for a particular number or letter, so using a color pattern to teach language often does not work as the colors are confused by each person's different color patterns. There are probably just as many color patterns and ways of "seeing" letters and numbers as there are colors and persons with synesthesia! Moreover, synesthesia shows how very subjective our world really is, and how many ways there are to perceive that subjectivity.

In her book, Duffy says that New York City Ballet composer Michael Torke uses colors in his compositions, which are his own synthetic creations, but sometimes wonders if the audience appreciates his music or if they are responding to the intriguing colors (81). This is a creative decision that many artists who also have synesthesia must contend with. Many synesthetes also employ the use of transforming, which is the process of changing one sensory creation into another, such as mathematical equations into colors (101). Many neuroscientists, such as Richard Cytowic, believe the limbic part of the brain is the seat of synesthesia, and that those with synesthesia are just more aware of their unconscious processes than those without the trait, due to different parts of the brain being disconnected from others (103).

Synesthetes can sometimes evoke deeper states of consciousness, as they can be in touch with their more subjective and hidden levels of awareness. Those that have a deeper connection with their inner worlds sometimes experience conflict with their outer worlds (116). The more attention that is paid to certain abstract signals from the unconscious, the more creative and artistic that unconscious consciousness seems to be. The dreams of some synesthetes are shown to be in totally different colors as well; they share the same components with language integration and colors (120).

Duffy lists the seven forms of intelligence: intrapersonal, which the artist Alfred Kubin possesses, interpersonal, kinesthetic, spatial, math/logical, linguistic, and musical (137). Mr. Kubin was not very good at math, but excelled in art, and could express his own synesthetic concurrents, or responses, through his internal processes. The way a particular person decodes information is unique, and the actual decoding itself is unique. Having this kind of perception helps synesthetes discover new information and forms a pathway for new creative endeavors, led by synesthesia (146). These are the building blocks of eidetic memory, where a sensation is not only seen by the visual preceptors, but also felt, as a sensation, within the body (142). Even for those who have day, month, and year maps, the perception of the time sequencing can be quite subjective. Some grapheme color synesthetes do not just see colors when they are given a letter stimulus, but they also perceive spatial and time sequencing (150). Moreover, Duffy states that Sean Day, PhD, synesthete, and who currently teaches anthropology, contends that synesthesia should be studied in order to learn more about the brain (161). Professor Day runs an email list (found at daysyn.com) for researchers, artists and synesthetes interested in learning more about synesthesia.

In *The Hidden Sense*, Cretien van Campen (2010) illustrates how math calculations are done by synesthetes who associate colors with numbers. The interesting fact about this is that this sensory connection is bi-directional, meaning it goes both ways. Colors are also used in calculating numbers, and vice versa. Indeed, numbers, days of the week, and months of the year can also be seen in spatial forms, sometimes called "visual thinking" (van Campen, 84). Albert Einstein said he would solve puzzles using this kind of thinking. Sometimes artists will discover different hidden forms of meaning through their first synthetic impressions.

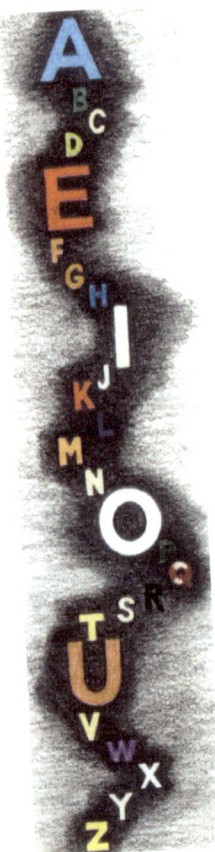

Figure 8   Retgien, 2007. Alphabet Colors and Spatial Forms.

The development of language is what separates the five conscious senses into different channels. In the 1980s, seven more senses were identified: movement, equilibrium, temperature, speech, imagination, life, and self (100). All of these senses were integrated. The Desana Indians' color energies were all wholly integrated: if one sense was stimulated, the rest were all affected (101).

Van Campen says that the three characteristics of color in synesthesia are tone, saturation, and lightness. While color was once thought to be universal, is now known that color is not always present in synesthesia as evidenced by congenitally blind synesthetes with sound to touch or flavor to sound synesthesia (Day, 2024). Those who develop true synesthesia have their own personal color systems and rely on internal mechanisms rather than on external ones (148).

CHAPTER 6

My Synesthesia

This author has grapheme color synesthesia. I have had it as long as I can remember, from the time I was in kindergarten. It has influenced how I learned to memorize days of the week, months of the year, numbers, the alphabet, you name it. Everything has always displayed itself in color. I see a color before I remember a name. My number colors are as follows:

1 = white, 2 = navy blue, 3 = sea green, 4 = shades of bright pink, but ranging from violet to light pink, 5 = purplish-navy blue, 6 = yellow, 7 = orange, 8 = dark green, 9 = brown, 10 = white and gray (0 = gray), 11 = double white, 12 = white and sea green, and so on, all through the double- and triple-digit numbers. When I think of numbers, I do not see a line necessarily, just the number symbols in their respective colors in my mind's eye. Because I don't see them in a spatial form, there is no far away or close up, they are just there.

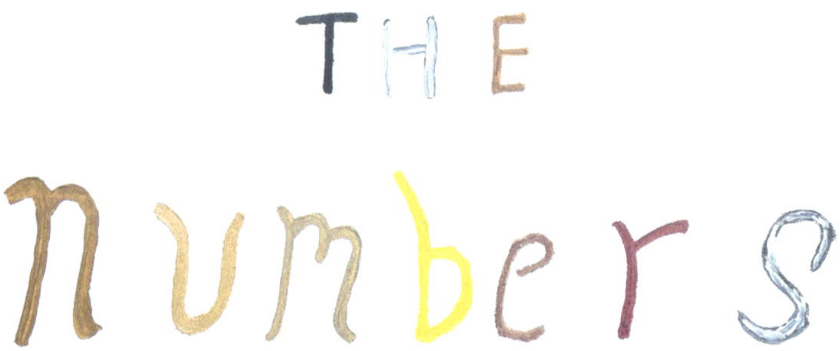

Figure 9   Rook, E.T. 2022. The Numbers Spelled Out.

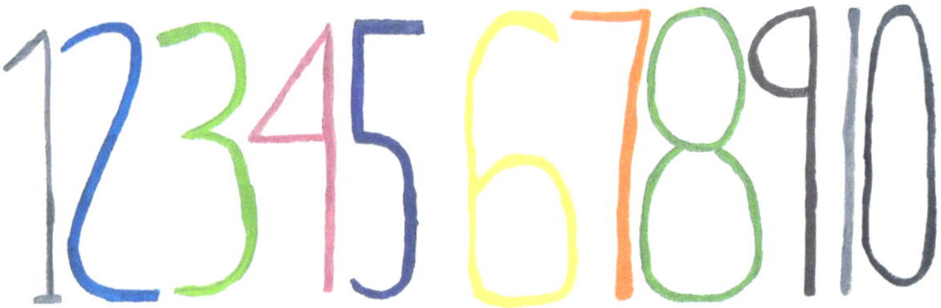

Figure 10   Rook, E.T. 2022. The Numbers, Digits.

However, for the days of the week, I see the seven names in a line, starting with Sunday, which is a deep violet; Monday is navy blue; Tuesday ranges from a hot pink to a bright red; Wednesday is red, but a bit darker than Tuesday; Thursday is dark green; Friday is bright yellow; and Saturday is light green. The colors of the names do not have anything to do with the individual letters that make up the names. The first letter of each name does not determine the day's color, in this case. But each name of the day has a dimension and a form; they are all rectangular shaped, sitting right next to each other, as if on a line.

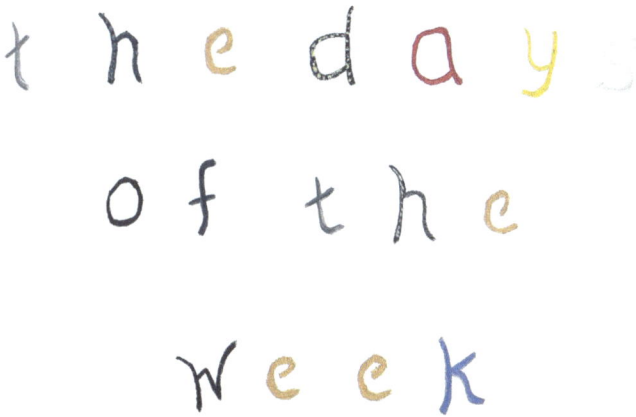

Figure 11   Rook, E.T. 2022. The Days of the Week (Text).

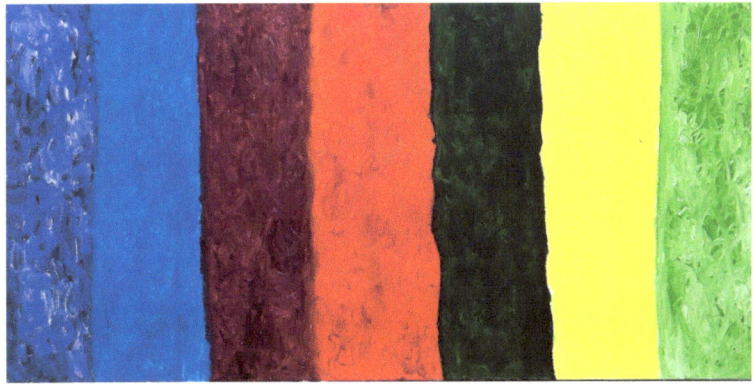

Figure 12   Rook, E.T. 2022. The Days of the Week (Colors).

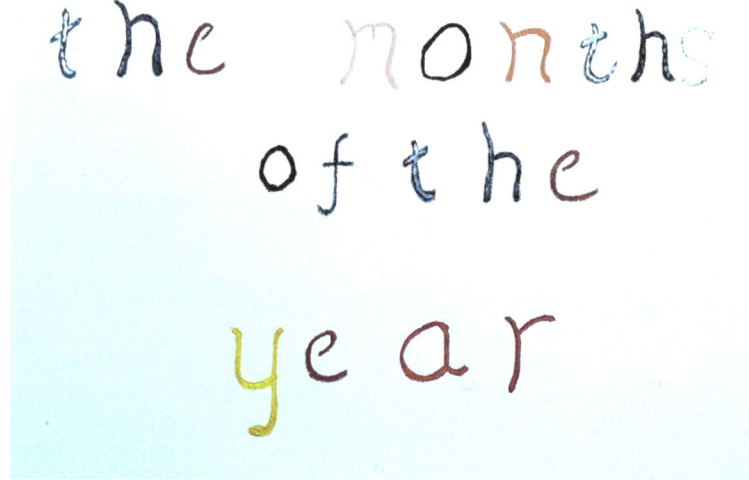

Figure 13   Rook, E.T. 2022. The Months of the Year (Text)

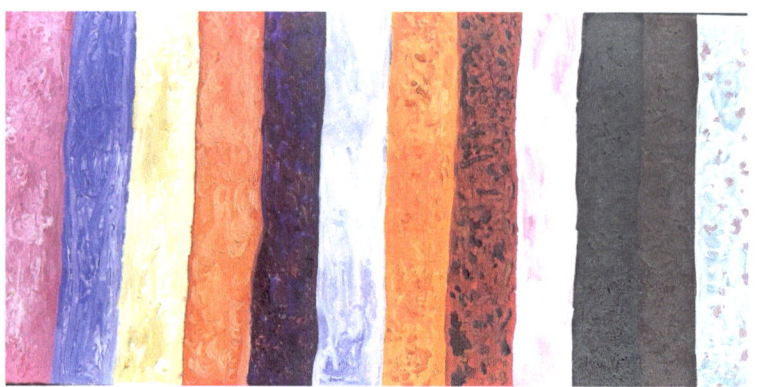

Figure 14   Rook, E.T. 2022. The Months of the Year (Colors)

The months of the year are similarly shaped to the days of the week. There is a rectangular form, and they are spaced closely together. January is a mix of red, pink, and white; it's as if it's not just one tone of color, but made up of three separate ones. February is like an amethyst; it can be lavender, violet, mauve, or dark purple, and it sparkles. March is mostly white with a bit of light green and maybe a hint of gold flecks. April is a red shade with light pink; May is a dark lavender; June is a light lavender; July is bright orange; August is purple with red and brown; September is pink with a little tan; October is black; November is brown; and December is mostly white and gray. I have no idea how I came up with these exact colors. All I know is that I've had them from the age of four or five, and they have been consistent throughout my life.

Now we come to individual words. With my grapheme color synesthesia, vowels have more color and are more dominant than consonants. This is the case for a lot of synesthetes with this type of synesthesia. Most vowels within the words "color" the color of the word itself. For instance, with the word "apple," the "a" is red; the "p" is gray, or a combination of black and white; "l" is only a very light lavender; and "e" is slightly tan, with a little rust. As the "a" is bright red, it controls the color of the word, and "apple" is mostly red. In the word "underwear," because the "u" is a golden, yellowish color with a bit of orange, the word "underwear" is mostly that color, as the "n" is light brown, "d" is black, "e" is tan, "r" is gold with a bit of orange, "w" is black, "e" is tan, "a" is red, and "r" is gold-orange. But the other colors are muted by the "u" color. The "e" and "a" stand out, and when I see the word in my mind's eye, I see the red and the tan of the "a" and the "e," but the primary color is the "u" color, which, although not strong, is a greenish-yellow. Most words are made up of both vowels and consonants, and there are very few words that have either one or the other. So, in any given word, with my synesthesia type, the vowels in that word control the color of the word. But what about a word that has a lot of vowels, such as "umbrella"?

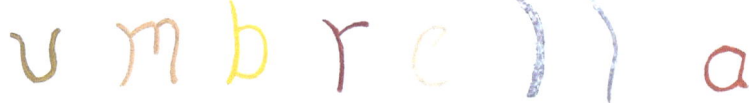

Figure 15   Rook, E.T. 2022. Umbrella.

Like with "underwear," the "u," which happens to also be the first letter, dominates the color of that word. The "m" is tan or neutral; "b," although normally yellow, is somewhat muted; "r" is golden; "e" is tan; "l" is gray-lavender; and "a," the last letter of the word, is red, but does not control the word's color, as it is the last phoneme on the word. Generally, the first letter controls the color of the word. What about a word that starts with a consonant, even two consonants, such as "chloroform"?

That word has a very dull color, as "c" is white, "h" is black, "l" is only a light lavender, "o" is black, "r" is gold but not strong enough to overpower the dull sheen of the overall word, "f" is black, and "m" is tannish. So the overall color of "chloroform" is black, or at best, a dark gray.

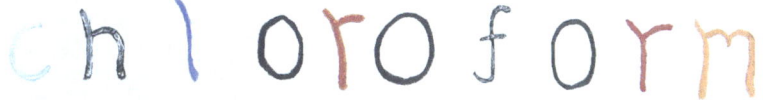

Figure 16   Rook, E.T. 2022. Chloroform.

The word "spinning" starts with two consonants, both of which are not very colorful letters. But the "i" is yellow-white, and there are two of them in "spinning," so that's a double whammy of yellow. "N" is just brownish-yellow, and "g" is bright, too, as golden orange, but because it's the last letter in the word, its color does not overpower the yellow of the "i," therefore, "spinning" is yellow.

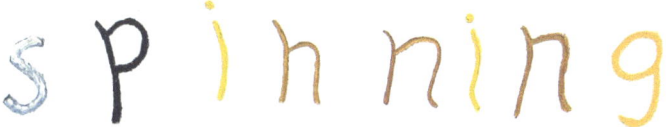

Figure 17   Rook, E.T. 2022. Spinning.

In phoneme color synesthesia, sounds are connected to different colors. However, as this author does not have this kind of synesthesia, phonemes are not a concern. This type of synesthesia is common, and many who have it associate specific colors with the sounds of letters. For example, each letter represents a different color, so for the words "pat" and "pad," the different letters "t" and "d" cause a resulting different color due to the differences in their sounds. In my case of grapheme synesthesia, the differing letters represent different colors.

In the case of homonyms, where a word sounds exactly the same but is spelled differently, grapheme color synesthesia kicks in. For example, the words "break" and "brake" are technically homophones because they sound the same, but have different spellings, and mean two totally different things. The letters making up the words are different as well. "Breaks" is color, because it has two vowels, "e" and" a," which are dominant and sort of share the color tan and red, so the word "break" is tannish-red. The word "brake," which has the same two vowels, is mostly a red word. The consonants in both "break" and "brake" are muted by the vowels. In the word "break," the "k" is the only consonant that has a slight effect on the entire word, a bluish purple, at the end of the word. But the "k" in "brake" does not affect the entire word's color as much as it has an "e" at the end.

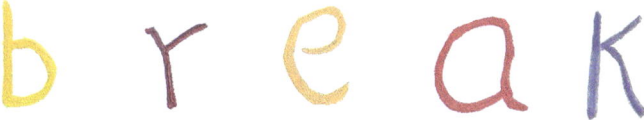

Figure 18   Rook, E.T. 2022. Break.

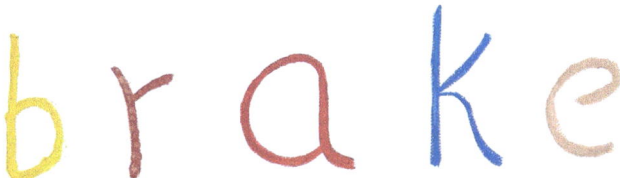

Figure 19   Rook, E.T. 2022. Brake.

The following is a mind's eye view of what my internal grapheme color scheme looks like for the days of the week. Oddly enough, certain words do have a visual-taste connection with my synesthesia. I was not really that aware of this until I realized that visual-taste synesthesia, or gustatory synesthesia, existed. Days of the week, months of the year, numbers, and the alphabet are all tied to a certain gustatory image. Almost all words, if I think long enough, can be associated with food with my synesthesia. As stated above, Sunday is dark purple with a bit of red marbling and is cold and sweet like ice cream; Monday is a dark navy blue and feels like canvas, but the associated food is navy bean soup; Tuesday is a mix of red shading with hot pink, and reminds me of tomato soup; Wednesday is mostly a dark red, and also reminds me of beef stew, with that same sort of consistency; Thursday is dark green, and I think of green vegetables, like broccoli or squash; Friday is yellow and feels/tastes like tortilla chips or popcorn; and Saturday is a light green, and doesn't really have a food connected with it, but I think of the ocean when it is choppy and looks sea green.

My January is mainly soft white but with little flecks of red and light pink, and the word reminds me of strawberry cream in the middle of chocolate candies. February is quite similar, and the word reminds me of the consistency of cherry cream inside chocolate-covered cherries, but the color is darker, almost a purple, with more blue swirls, creating a soft violet color. March is a huge departure from the first two months; it's a muted white, or beige-white, with bits of gold and yellow, but mostly white. Even though the letters that make up March have little yellow or white (they are actually fairly neutral), and the "a" is red, the color of the month is different. The food it reminds me of is hard to define; it is soft, salty, and starchy, like bread or macaroni. April is back to the red, orange, warm shades, with just a touch of cream, but not much. April's food is apricots, very similar to the colors of the letter, and the sound of the word. May is a dark purple, or lavender shade, and is sweet and syrupy. June is a light lavender with a tart but sweet taste, and I'm not sure exactly what food it is, but like May, it is syrupy. July is bright orange and is the brightest color of any month of the year in my color inventory. July has always reminded me of orange slices, those jelly candies that are supposed to resemble fruit, and are covered in sugar. August is a darker mauve, purple, color but follows the previous months in the sweet category. Another fruity, sugar dripping word that is on the jelly candy list. September changes a bit with lighter shades of white and pink, and is not really associated with food of any kind, just a pinkish hue and has a soft, malleable texture. Sort of like icing on a cake … maybe mine, as it is my birthday month. In October, as "o" is black, the month is blacker than black. There is no food associated with October either, not in the sense of synesthesia of the grapheme color kind. November is like October, but the color of November is a dark brown, and there is little taste, or food connected to this month as well. Again, December has no food, except perhaps ice, and the color of December is white, with a little blue gray mixed in. Sorry, no red and green here!

Do numbers have tastes/foods associated with them? The answer is yes, they do, but some are stronger than others.

#0 is gray, and does not have a very strong taste or food, but if I had to say, it would be close to a baked potato, with the same soft, crumbly consistency.

#1 is white, like mayonnaise.

#2 is navy blue, and is similar to chicken broth, or any warm liquid with a salty taste.

#3 is light green and could be close to a vegetable, with the same color hue, such as lettuce, or watercress.

#4 is pinkish red and its associated food/taste is a sweet sugary substance, such as red licorice.

#5 is violet, and this is associated with any dark berry, such as blueberries, and often the crust of a blueberry pie is included.

#6 is yellow and is salty and crunchy, like potato chips, popcorn, or tortilla chips.

#7 is orange and is any tangy food, such as oranges, grapefruit, or fruit juice, mainly orange or anything with an acidic flavor.

#8 is dark green and is usually associated with dark leafy green vegetables, such as broccoli, spinach, or kale.

#9 is brown and could be beef gravy, as it has the same consistency and texture as this savory accompaniment to meat.

#10 is white and gray, similarly, and is close to a meat—it could be beef.

#11 is double white and is very much like chicken gravy because of the color and texture.

#12 is white and navy blue and so on, and so forth, as the colors of the number form play out. For some reason, #12 reminds me of ham, not sure exactly how, but that is the mystery of synesthesia. I could go on and on with all the numbers, listing their colors and the associated tastes of each, all the way up to #100, but I have already named the individual colors of each number #1-10, and their colors. The foods of each number are different, and totally unpredictable, unlike the colors after #9. I will list my associated tastes/foods from the number #13-25 for your reference here, but for the sake of time and space, I will stop there.

To continue:

#13 is white and light green. It has the consistency of celery.

#14 is red and white and could be a lot of different things, but is mainly sweet, red, and white-colored candy, like peppermint sticks.

#15 is white and purple, and is a berry pastry, like #5, such as blueberry pie.

#16 is white and yellow and has a salty taste; it could be any kind of chips.

#17 is orange and white and has tangerine or orange flavors.

#18 is white and dark forest green, and anything that is green in color, even a fruit is possible, like pears or green grapes.

#19 is white and brown, and tastes like anything that is brown, like gravy or some kind of beef.

#20 is navy blue and gray and has a very liquid, soupy texture.

#21 is white and dark blue, and the food is a combination of mayonnaise and chicken soup, or even a lunch meat such as ham or salami.

#22 is double navy blue and is either like chicken soup or a liquid, salty mixture.

#23 is navy blue and light green, and is a soup made of vegetables.

#24 is dark blue and reddish/pink with no real food or taste associated with it because I can't think of any that matches blue and red.

#25 is dark blue and purple, and again, there is no clear-cut food associated with it, only the remnants of the blueberry.

From here, the tastes remain the same for all the numbers, with just the remnants of the blueberry. Also, the first number in the sequence is not as dominant as the rest of the numbers contained within the number. The last number in the number sequence is most dominant and determines its color and/or food taste. But the higher the numbers go, the more complicated or nuanced the colors get, and the food associated is usually the last number in the sequence. For example, with #412, the "4" is red, the "1" is white, and the "2" is dark blue, so there is no clear food or taste. This is true for all numbers through infinity.

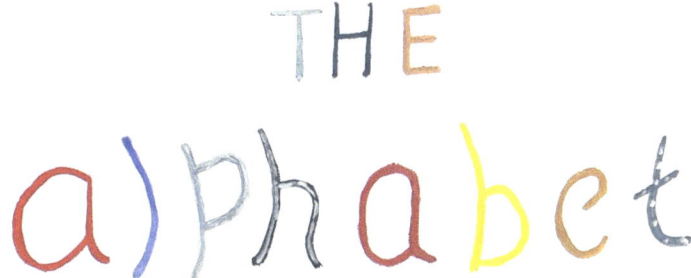

Figure 20   Rook, E.T.2022. The Alphabet (Text).

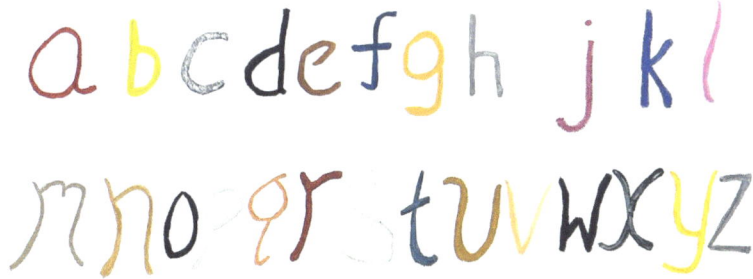

Figure 21   Rook, E.T. 2022. The Alphabet (Colors).

The food and color associations of the alphabet, like the numbers, are mainly in the mind's eye. There is not a clear-cut line of letters, but when I visualize them, I can see the entire alphabet from left to right. I can also see them separately and individually.

Now this author will discuss the letters of the alphabet. The letter "a" is red, and reminds me of apples, or anything slightly sweet;

"b" is yellow, and is like some kind of smooth pasta, like in alphabet soup;

"c" is white-gray, and really does not have a food or taste association;

"d" is grayish-black and is sort of like "b" in that it has a pasta associated with it, like macaroni;

"e" is tannish-brown, and its food association is ground beef;

"f" is grayish-black and reminds me of a kids' cereal, like Lucky Charms, and must be something soft and chewy;

"g" is goldish-orange, and is a kind of cheese, or could be any soft cheese, like Swiss or Gruyere;

"h" is blackish-gray and does not have a strong food associated with it;

"i" is white and its food association is milk;

"j" has grayish-lavender undertones and reminds me of another type of cereal, like Cheerios or Apple Jacks;

"k" is dark blue-purple, similar to the #5 and connotes a sweet taste, such as cake;

"i" is a lighter shade of lavender, mixed with a bit of gray, and reminds me of a soft, watery food like milk;

"m" is yellowish-tan, and could be a type of pasta, or even be similar to a garbanzo bean;

"n" is a creamy color, with a bit of brown, and similar to a kind of nut;

"o" is black and does not have a strong food associated with it;

"p" is whitish-gray, and is like cotton, with no food association;

"q" is a golden-orangish-rust color, and almost reminds me of honey;

"r" is similar to "q" with all the same color tones, but is just a few shades darker and like a kind of candy, such as Butterfingers;

"s" is grayish-white, and does not have a food or taste associated with it;

"t" is like "s" and is only a few shades darker, and has no food associated with it;

"u" is a dark amber color with mustard yellow, and a bit of orange, and is similar to mustard;

"v" is like "m" with a tannish color and is associated with pasta;

"w" is gray-black, and does not have a strong food association;

"x" is grayish-black like "w," but is a bit lighter in shade, and does not have a food association;

"y" is yellow-white, and is associated with butter, or something creamy, like gravy;

and lastly, "z" is a gray-blue, and is not associated with a food.

One type of synesthesia, which has not been fully discussed here yet, is where letters and numbers take on personality types, or even texture/aroma types. I never really thought much about whether I had this kind, but upon reading and researching about it, I suppose I do.

The following list is my personality/texture/gender/aroma types for numbers up to #20, and for the alphabet.

#1 cool, determined, orderly, male, creamy
#2 fluid, smart, female, watery
#3 fun-loving, very likeable, male or female, aromatic
#4 female, happy, light-hearted, sweet
#5 male, rich, touchy-feely, juicy
#6 female, sporty, active, salty
#7 male, intelligent, academic, acidy
#8 female, artistic, creative, herbaceous
#9 likes the outdoors, female, soupy
#10 mundane, male, spongy but strong
#11 uniform, neutral, male, creamy

#12 male, smart, well rounded, tough but malleable

#13 male or female, very relaxed, loose, easygoing, crunchy

#14 female, likes to cook, very domestic, flavorful

#15 male, open, does not take a lot of chances, crusty

#16 female, active, athletic, savory

#17 male, caring, heart of gold, energizing

#18 female, outgoing, versatile, jelly

#19 male, nerdy, likes to play chess, globby

#20 male, smart, bookworm, fluid

Alphabet

A, a, tart, female, apple scent

B, b, sassy, outgoing, female, chewy

C, c, boring, male, smooth

D, d, unpleasant, female, round, and hard

E, e, female, friendly, semi-solid

F, f, male-dark, cereal

G, g, female happy, cheesy

H, h, male smooth talker, airy

I, i, male true, loyal, milky

J, j male, good sense of humor, crunchy

K, k, female, malleable, cakey

L, l, female, sweet-natured, drippy

M, m, female, open, well-rounded, soft

N, n, male protector, rough

O, o, female, feminine, warm

P, p, female, punctual, cottony

Q, q, female, different, honey

R, r, female, fun-loving, candy-like

S, s, female, flexible, balloon-like

T, t, male, strong, steely

U, u, male, covert, mustard-like

V, v, male, unyielding, spongy

W, w, male, jack of all trades, rubbery

X, x, male, constant, invisible

Y, y, male, motherly, buttery

Z, z male, skeptical, tinny

For the most part, colors are the most conscious part of my synesthesia. These colors relate to the alphabet and numbers, including days of the week, and months of the year. But if I think about it, I also associate personalities and textures with the letters and numbers, as indicated above. I suppose that these lesser associations are less conscious in my brain than the colors of numbers and letters, and probably formed later. Also, each individual letter of a word has a color, but the entire word itself also has a color. It sounds confusing, but it is not when you have synesthesia. It's like an amazing puzzle you hold the solution to, like there is an automatic map inside your head of every word, every letter in the universe, and nothing can change that.

Trying to remember a person's name is easy because I can remember what color that person's name was. Usually their name is on the tip of my tongue once I remember the color. And of course, synesthetes' colors are deeply nuanced, and there can be many shades of one color. The differing shades of colors are what make up the synesthete's mind/color map and there are as many shades and hues of a color as there are synesthetes to see them.

I suppose I could think of colors when I hear sound, or musical notes, but I don't think I have hearing color synesthesia, nor do I have touch synesthesia. The colors must be completely automatic when a sound is given, and for me that does not happen as easily with sounds.

CHAPTER 7
Experiments in Synesthesia

In this chapter, different experiments, both artistic and psychological in synesthesia, will be discussed. As mentioned in Chapter 2, color and pitch were the subject of much experimentation, as the two senses were thought to be related in synesthesia. In the online article "Artistic and Psychological Experiments with Synesthesia" (1999), Cretien van Campen states the Greek mathematician Pythagoras related both pitch and color, but there was no system of correlation between the two senses. Newton finally discovered that light waves could be this system of correlation, and in 1720, Castel invented a harpsichord with a system of lights that lit up when a sound or key was heard or pressed. Scriabin contended that changing the color of the musical composition when the tonality changed would be "a powerful psychological resonator for the listener," as opposed to changes with the change in tone alone. Technical problems marred his first performance, and subsequent performances using this technique failed due to other reasons, even after Scriabin's death, through no fault of Scriabin's.

As music was regarded as the highest level of art, during this time, because it could not be seen, visual art was regarded as being a lower form of artistic expression on the scale. In the late 19th century, visual art was combined with music, and artist groups started to flourish that combined different arts. Kandinsky started experimenting with unifying the artistic experience with dancers, theatrical producers, musicians, and artists who joined their artistic expressions into one main composition or performance. The concepts of dissonance, along with consonance, were also the target of experimentation, resulting in what the composers hoped would have a "deeper impact." With the addition of physical and visual dissonance, the artist hoped to give the audience a much improved and stronger experience with the arts, and paved the way for more experimentation in the Gestalt and emotional aspects of synesthesia in the mid-20th century. Many symbolists, such as Kandinsky himself, believed in the early 20th century that music was on a higher level than art. Kandinsky wrote *The Spiritual in Art*, which marked a turning point in the development of art within music, and the search for a higher artistic expression in painting (57).

Dutch artist Piet Mondrian wanted to introduce more fluidity into what was considered at the time to be static art. The concept of movement was studied and, in Mondrian's *Composition with Gray Lines*, a series of grids was etched into a rhombus type shape with different thicknesses of lines. The idea of movement and, therefore, a fourth dimension of time, was added to the other three dimensions of an artist's canvas. Most of the experiments, however, gave mixed results, and the conclusion was that the idea of time and movement in art was never fully realized. Mondrian applied more depth to art by applying different visual grids, allowing the paintings to become less static and to be on a level with the depth of musical expression. Additionally, current experiments with sound and color seem to focus more on the physics of synesthesia, rather than the psychological aspects which were the focus of past experiments through Scriabin, Kandinsky, and Mondrian.

Early on, synesthesia was thought to be an abnormal functioning of the brain, but with time and experimentation, that concept gradually lessened. By the 19th century, most believed synesthesia was a normal part of cognitive functioning that was more developed in some than others. Fechner conducted the first organized study of the psychological aspects of synesthesia on seventy-three subjects, and by the psychologist Marks on four hundred subjects. Nothing of great importance was discovered, except that with grapheme-color synesthesia, bright consonants corresponded with light colors, and dark ones with dark colors. Laboratory experiments with subjects emerged in the 1920s, and these experiments focused on whether physiological mechanisms caused the origins of synesthesia or had their roots in the mental recollection of sense data.

More experiments with studying the unity of the senses were conducted by psychologists, such as Von Hornbostel and Werner. These experiments had subjects matching gray cards with differing odors. The subjects were then given a pitch that they were to match to a gray card. This experiment measured the sense modality of brightness, but did not consider other dimensions of touch or other senses, as brightness was assumed to be the unifying common sense within the total senses. After WWII, synesthesia was thought to be metaphor, and interest in experimenting with the traits waned. Since then, synesthesia has enjoyed more neuropsychological interest, and recent studies have started using more well-defined tests to determine synesthetes from non-synesthetes and more well-defined criteria. The most current thought on the trait is still a debate between the modularists and the unitarists. Modularists believe that synesthesia is caused by neural misfiring, and the unitarists believe it is caused by a natural emotional process centered in the limbic system.

For the most part, synesthesia is difficult to study and there are no hard and fast rules by which to understand the phenomenon. Artistic experiments have shown the dynamic aspects of synesthesia, and psychological ones have shown criteria for assessing it, and for the analysis of certain aspects of it.

In Simon Baron Cohen and John E. Harrison's book *Synesthesia: Classic and Contemporary Readings* (1997), the subject of learned association was tested with synesthetes who associated colors with letters, and with non-synesthetes who did not. Their brain patterns of cerebral blood flow are being compared as this book is written. Additionally, the acquisition of reading skills is also thought to shift between pre-reading, where the actual correspondence is based on phonology of a word, and post-reading, where the correspondence is based upon the spelling of the word (121). Synesthesia is a broad range of sense collaboration which can take years, if not decades, to research properly and develop conclusions.

For some synesthetes, the music of Prince induced different colors and patterns, depending on where the attention of the synesthete was located, such as whether they were focused on the sounds or the emotions of the music (Van Campen, 12). The triggers and concurrents can go in opposite directions, that is, sounds can induce colors, and colors can trigger sounds for some persons.

As noted in Cytowic's book, *The Man Who Tasted Shapes*, Michael Watson, a taste-touch-smell synesthete, experienced less strong synesthetic perceptions, such as the shapes or textures, when he drank caffeine, and stronger ones when he drank alcohol. This confirmed Cytowic's theory that synesthesia starts in the limbic system because he found that the cortex nearly shuts down during synesthetic perceptions (142).

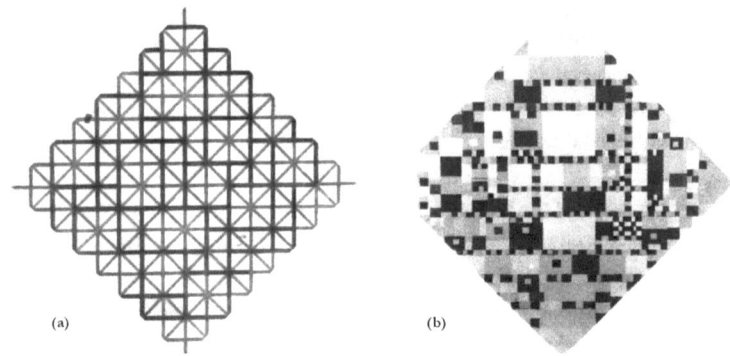

Figure 22   Mondrian, 1918, and 1942-1944.
Composition with Grey Lines and Victory Boogie Woogie.

In *Blue Cats and Chartreuse Kittens* by Patricia Lynne Duffy, the importance of the subjective over the objective is illustrated by the fact that doctors often make observations of patients' subjective experiences when making diagnoses, and drawing conclusions. Since the 1960s, when only objective reports were considered when examining the synesthesia phenomenon, the tide has turned back to observing more subjective accounts, and listening to the accounts of those with the trait (Duffy, 27).

With grapheme-color synesthesia, experiments were performed to illustrate that numbers are not perceived without their corresponding color. The grapheme does not have to be written or even spoken for the person to visualize the color that corresponds to it. Another experiment showed that numbers are not perceived apart from their colors, with numbers shown on different colored backgrounds (71).

CHAPTER 8

Personal Accounts of Synesthesia

In this chapter, the author explores personal accounts of several people with synesthesia, and their differing types. One account involves Rainye Cole, a native Australian living in this country for a few years who experiences chromesthesia—seeing colors when music is played. Rianye also has colored perceptions when experiencing pain; the sensation is like an electrical shock, the color is a deep maroon red. For example, when sitting, the perception is like lightning that burns, and colors such as brown, maroon, and red streaks are perceived. Emotions are also involved—a form of synesthesia called associative synesthesia—the combination of the two is almost indescribable, according to him. Different songs bring out different types of emotions, and the emotions are experienced as colors. If the colors match the emotions of the music, then it's okay. Other perceptions involve seeing images with music, as well as colors. Rainye also can taste certain colors as well, known as visual-gustatory synesthesia.

The color blue evokes the taste of coconut; the color green evokes oranges; black, salt; orange, sour; brown, ginger; red, dust; purple, chocolate; and silver, apple juice.

The lyrics of a song induce colored letters, depending on the emotion of the lyrics.

Rainye writes a short essay on dealing with depression as colors are grounding, they help deal with emotions. We all have a destination and a purpose, the blogger states, and life is not about the destination but the journey. It is our quest to find out what that purpose is. The colors help in finding that peace and quiet within themselves. Some days are easier than others, but we must keep moving on, throughout the chaos and the darkness (Cole, 2020).

This next synesthete, Carla, has colored hearing with music and perception. She is also lexical-gustatory. The word *"propos"* in French to her brings on a taste of a sauce of tomatoes, basil, and Gruyere. The German language induces perceptions of cake batter. Some voices, like sounds, bring on flavors as well. This synesthete's sister has lexical-gustatory synesthesia also, with words having a taste. In a strange twist, their parents do not have it, as they are from dissimilar backgrounds (Carla, 2023).

The following synesthete says having synesthesia makes life worth living!!

Identified only by a Reddit handle, another synesthete, Cycleoverload, claims to have OCD (obsessive-compulsive disorder) patterns that match auditory or tactile sensations. Their numbers and letters have colors which makes math and memory very easy. Cycleoverload remembers numbers and words by flipping through an internal index and searching top to bottom. Sets of colors are used for passwords, like a rainbow or pride flag.

In proprioception, which is the ability to sense movement, or kinesthesia, Cycleoverload's mind and body makes a fog in the shape of all objects. Specific points can be searched for and details obtained from the object. Cycleoverload feels this and sees the details of the object.

Music can induce colors and shapes and overpower the fog. The fog does not have a shape. Sometimes Cycleoverload will fall when this happens because they are off balance. The difference between sound and word color is that sound color has meaning. Colors have emotion too—white is empty; black is powerful; pink is comforting; red is intense; orange is beautiful or unsettling; yellow is loving or smothering; green is confusion; blue is sad and cold; and purple is balance, like being cold and wet but wrapped in a towel. For Cycleoverload, voices and names have colors, and a person's color is different from their name solely (Cycleoverload, 2023).

Grapheme synesthete Alice S. says she did not realize she had grapheme synesthesia until she was 65. She is now 82 years old. Ms. Schultze was featured in *Tasting the Universe*, by Maureen Seaberg. This synesthete, a writer, did not realize there was a name for her trait. She also mused on synesthesia and spirituality, thinking that there must be some connection but never being exactly sure how they were entwined. (Schultze, 2023.)

Another synesthete, Robin P., has lexical-gustatory synesthesia. This synesthete senses taste when seeing or hearing words, sounds, shapes, colors, and movement. Robin was not aware that synesthesia had a name until much older. When a child, Robin said friends thought it strange that their names had a taste. This synesthete received two scholarships to university, and was accepted into a well-known music conservatory. Possessing a photographic memory, this synesthete experienced trauma as a child and does not know if that was a factor in the synesthetic perception. Robin is currently a mosaic artist. Neither the parents nor the sons of Robin are synesthetes. (Peckover, 2023).

Acknowledgements

No book is ever written without a list of those who have helped in creating a dream for the author. This effort was certainly one of those. I wish to acknowledge my husband, first and foremost, Roger, who is always there for support in any literary endeavor I may take on. Secondly, I thank both my boys, Wiley and Kirby, for always being supportive as well, and to Wiley, especially, for his artistic support in his beautiful and creative works for *Sense and Synesthesia.*

I thank my editor, Joanne, from Firstediting whom I have used for the last two books I have written, and the whole team, for their constant and unwavering input and professionalism in the editing of this book. Thank you to MIT Press, specifically Pamela Quick, for granting permission to use material from the Press. Thank you to the folks at Copyright Clearance Center for assistance with the other permissions in this book.

Thank you to Sean Day, for his guidance and input in the overall factual information for this book and his support.

Lastly, I wish to thank Kate Winter, with From Manuscript to Book, for assisting in the amalgamation of all of the various parts of *Sense and Synesthesia* into a completed whole, making my dream a reality.

BIBLIOGRAPHY

Bender, Aimee. 2010. *The Particular Sadness of Lemon Cake: A Novel.* New York: Anchor.

Cytowic, Richard E., M.D. 2018. *Synesthesia.* Cambridge: MIT Press.

Cytowic, Richard E., M.D. 2008. *The Man Who Tasted Shapes, Revised Edition.* Cambridge: MIT Press.

Cytowic, Richard E., M.D, and David M. Eagleman. 2009. *Wednesday Is Indigo Blue: Discovering the Brain of Synesthesia.* Cambridge: MIT Press.

Duffy, Patricia Lynne. 2001. *Blue Cats and Chartreuse Kittens: How Synesthetes Color Their Worlds.* London: Macmillan.

Harrison, John E. and Simon Baron-Cohen. 1997. *Synaesthesia: Classic and Contemporary Readings.* Hoboken: Wiley-Blackwell.

Leatherdale, Lyndsay. 2013. *Synesthesia. The Fascinating World of Blended Senses. Synesthesia and Types of Synesthesia Explained. Tests, Symptoms, Causes and Treatment Options Al.* IMB Publishing.

Mass, Wendy. 2005. *A Mango-Shaped Space.* Boston: Little, Brown Books for Young Readers.

Moss, Laura. 2020. "Synesthesia." *Psychology Today.*

van Campen, Cretien. 2010. *The Hidden Sense: Synesthesia in Art and Science.* Cambridge: MIT Press.

Wikipedia. "Synesthesia." Wikimedia Foundation. Last modified 15 October 2023. https://en.wikipedia.org/w/index.php?title=Synesthesia&oldid=907042713.

Wikipedia. "Autonomous Sensory Meridian Response." Wikimedia Foundation. Last modified 8 October 2019. https://en.wikipedia.org/w/index.php?title=Autonomous_sensory_meridian_response&oldid=920235386.

REFERENCES

Image 1

Mysid, 2007, Wikimedia Commons contributors, "File:Synesthesia.svg," Wikimedia Commons, modified September 6, 2023, https://commons.wikimedia.org/w/index.php?title=File:Synesthesia.svg&oldid=798898170 (accessed September 5, 2019)

Image 2

Galton,1881. "Galton Number Form," Wikipedia, last modified January 15, 2023, https://commons.wikimedia.org/w/index.php?title=File:Synesthesia.svg&oldid=725209306 (accessed09/19/23

Chapter 1

Cytowic, Richard E., M.D., and David M. Eagleman, Ph.D. afterword by Dmitri Nabokov. 2011. *Wednesday Is Indigo Blue. Discovering the Brain of Synesthesia*, p.1, 72, short text excerpt, © 2009. Massachusetts Institute of Technology, by permission of The MIT Press.

Cytowic, Richard E., M.D. 2018. *Synesthesia*, p.3, 15, 16, 20-28, short text excerpt, © 2018 Massachusetts Institute of Technology, by permission of The MIT Press.

Cytowic, Richard E. 1997. "Phenomenology and Neuropsychology, a Review of Current Knowledge." In *Synaesthesia: Classic and Contemporary Readings*, edited by Simon Baron-Cohen and John E. Harrison. p.17, 19, 24, 25, 38 Hoboken: Blackwell Publishing.

Day, Sean, email to author, 7 April 2024. Via Simner, Julia and Duncan A. Carmichael. 2015. "Is Synesthesia a Dominantly Female Trait?" *Cognitive Neuroscience*, Vol. 6 (2-3): 68-76.

Harrison, John E. and Simon Baron-Cohen. 1997. "A Review of Psychological Theories." In *Synesthesia: Classic and Contemporary Readings*, edited by Simon Baron-Cohen and John E. Harrison, p.115. Hoboken: Blackwell Publishing.

Leatherdale, Lindsay. 2013. *Synesthesia: The Fascinating World of Blended Senses*, p.11,42, IMB Publishing.

Moss, Laura. "Synesthesia." *Psychology Today*. 13 February 2020.

http://www.laurajmoss.com/wp-content/uploads/2020/06/synesthesia.pdf.

van Campen, Cretien. 2010. *The Hidden Sense: Synesthesia in Art and Science*. p.124, 127, short text excerpt. @2010.Massachussetts institute of Technology, by permission of the MIT Press. MIT Press.

Wikipedia contributors, "Synesthesia," Wikipedia. Modified 15 October 2023. Accessed 20 July 2019. https://en.wikipedia.org/w/index.php?title=Synesthesia&oldid=907042713.

Image 3

Cytowic, Richard E., M.D. "Kluver's Form Constants," *Wednesday Is Indigo Blue*, figure 8.1 page 164, Cambridge: © 2008 Massachusetts Institute of Technology, by permission of MIT Press.

Chapter 2

Cytowic, Richard E., M.D., and David M. Eagleman, Ph.D. afterword by Dmitri Nabokov, *Wednesday Is Indigo Blue. Discovering the Brain of Synesthesia*, p.68,133, short text excerpt, Cambridge: © 2009 Massachusetts Institute of Technology, by permission of The MIT Press.

Cytowic, Richard E., M.D, 2018. *Synesthesia*, p.60,66, 67, 107, 127, 129, 143,161,164, short text excerpt: @2018 Massachusetts Institute of Technology, by permission of MIT Press.

Leatherdale, Lindsay. 2013. *The Fascinating World of Blended Senses*, p.9, IMB Publishing.

Marks, Lawrence. 1997. "On Colored Hearing Synesthesia; Cross Modal Translations of Sensory Dimensions." In *Synesthesia: Classic and Contemporary Readings*, edited by Simon Baron-Cohen and John E. Harrison, p.57, 71, 75, Hoboken: Blackwell Publishing.

Wikipedia contributors, "Autonomous Sensory Meridian Response," Wikipedia, October 8, 2019. https://en.wikipedia.org/w/index.php?title=Autonomous_sensory_meridian_response&oldid=920235386

Wikipedia contributors, "Synesthesia," Wikipedia, last modified 14 August 2023, accessed July 3, 2022. https://en.wikipedia.org/w/index.php?title=Synesthesia&oldid=1095743954.

Chapter 3

Cohut, Maria, Ph.D. "Synesthesia: Hearing Colors and Tasting Sounds." *Medical News Today,* August 17, 2018. https://www.medicalnewstoday.com/articles/322807.php.

Critchley, Edmund M. R. 1997. "Possible Mechanisms." In *Synesthesia: Classic and Contemporary Readings*, p.260, edited by Simon Baron-Cohen and John E. Harrison. Hoboken: Blackwell Publishing.

Cytowic, Richard E., M.D. foreword by Jonathan Cole, *The Man Who Tasted Shapes*; p.126,135.150,163,203, short text excerpt, © 2003 Massachusetts Institute of Technology, by permission of The MIT Press.

Cytowic, Richard E., M.D., and David M. Eagleman, Ph.D. afterword by Dmitri Nabokov, 2011. *Wednesday Is Indigo Blue. Discovering the Brain of Synesthesia*, p.77, 94, short text excerpt, © 2009 Massachusetts Institute of Technology, by permission of The MIT Press.

Cytowic, Richard E., M.D., *Synesthesia*, p.211,212, short text excerpt, © 2018 Massachusetts Institute of Technology, by permission of The MIT Press.

Day, Sean, PhD. Email to author. 7 April 2024.

Price, Michael. "Synaesthesia's Mysterious 'Mingling of the Senses' May Result from Hyperconnected Neurons." *Science*. March 5, 2018. https://www.science.org/content/article/synesthesia-s-mysterious-mingling-senses-may-result-hyperconnected-neurons

van Campen, Cretien, The Hidden Sense; p.113, short text excerpt, © 2008 Massachusetts Institute of Technology, by permission of The MIT Press.

Image 4

Cytowic, Richard E.M.D. foreword by Jonathan Cole, *The Man Who Tasted Shapes*, The Triune Brain, figure 2, p 21; © 2003 Massachusetts Institute of Technology, by permission of The MIT Press.

Chapter 4

Baron-Cohen, Simon and John Harrison. 1997. "Synesthesia: A Review of Psychological Theories." In *Synesthesia: Classic and Contemporary Readings*, p.110,112,114,115,116, 117, edited by Simon Baron-Cohen and John E. Harrison. Hoboken: Blackwell Publishing.

Cytowic, Richard E., M.D., and David M. Eagleman, Ph.D. afterword by Dmitri Nabokov, *Wednesday Is Indigo Blue. Discovering the Brain of Synesthesia*, p.243, short text excerpt, © 2009 Massachusetts Institute of Technology, by permission of The MIT Press.

Cytowic, Richard E., M.D. foreword by Jonathan Cole, *The Man Who Tasted Shapes*, p.20,76,91, short text excerpt, © 2003 Massachusetts Institute of Technology, by permission of The MIT Press.

Day, Sean, PhD. Email to author. 7 April 2024.

Frith, Christopher D. and Eraldo Paulescu. 1997. "The Physiological Basis of Synesthesia." In *Synesthesia: Classic and Contemporary Readings*, p.125, 128, 143, edited by Simon Baron-Cohen and John E. Harrison. Hoboken: Blackwell Publishing.

Grossenbacher, Peter. 1997. "Perception and Sensory Information in Synesthetic Experience." In *Synesthesia: Classic and Contemporary Readings*, p.155, 161, edited by Simon Baron-Cohen and John E. Harrison. Hoboken: Blackwell Publishing.

Maurer, Daphne. 1997. "Neonatal Synesthesia: Implications for the Processing of Faces and Speech." In *Synesthesia: Classic and Contemporary Readings*, p.225, 229, 236, edited by Simon Baron-Cohen and John E. Harrison. Hoboken: Blackwell Publishing.

Image 5

Rook, Wiley E. 2024. *Mango*.

Image 6

Rook, E, T. 2024. *Sweden and Thankfulness*.

Image 7

Rook, Wiley E. 2023. *Young Man Turning into a Chair*.

Image 8

van Campen, Cretien, *The Hidden Sense*, Katinka Retgien's Alphabet Color and Spatial Forms. Plate 1, page 93, © 2008 Massachusetts Institute of Technology, by permission of The MIT Press.

Chapter 5

Bender, Aimee. 2011. *The Particular Sadness of Lemon Cake*. New York: First Anchor Books.

Day, Sean. Email message to author.7 April.2024 via Tomson, Steffie N., Nili Avidan, Kwanghyuk Lee, Anand K. Sarma, Rejnal Tushe, Dianna M. Milewicz, Molly Bray, Suzanne M. Leal, and David M. Eagleman. 2011. "The genetics of color sequence synesthesia: Suggestive evidence of linkage to 16q and genetic heterogeneity for the condition." *Behavioural Brain Research*; vol. 223: 48 - 52.

Duffy, Patricia Lynne. 2001. *Blue Cats and Chartreuse Kittens*, p.9, 28, 41, 54, 73, 81, 101, 103, 116, 120, 137, 142, 146, 150, 161, New York: Henry

Holt and Company.

Mass, Wendy. 2005. *A Mango-Shaped Space.* Boston: Little Brown and Company.

Motluck, Alison. 1997. "Two Synesthetes Talking Color." In *Synesthesia: Classic and Contemporary Readings,* edited by Simon Baron-Cohen and John E. Harrison. p.269-277. Hoboken: Blackwell Publishing.

van Campen, Cretien, *The Hidden Sense,* p.84,100,101,137,148, short text excerpt, © 2008 Massachusetts Institute of Technology, by permission of The MIT Press.

Image 9
  E. T. Rook, 2022, The Numbers Spelled Out.

Image 10
  E. T. Rook, 2022, The Numbers (digits).

Image 11
  E. T. Rook, 2022, The Days of the Week (text).

Image 12
  E. T. Rook, 2022, The Days of the Week (colors).

Image 13
  E. T. Rook, 2022, The Months of the Year, (text).

Image 14
  E. T. Rook, 2022, The Months of the Year (colors).

Image 15
  E. T. Rook, 2022, Umbrella.

Image 16
  E T Rook, 2022, Chloroform.

Image 17
  E. T. Rook, 2022, Spinning.

Image 18
  E. T. Rook, 2022, Break.

Image 19
    E T Rook, 2022, Brake.

Image 20
    E. T. Rook, 2022, The Alphabet.
Image 21
    E. T. Rook, 2022, The Alphabet (colors).

Image 22
    van Campen, Cretien, The Hidden Sense, *Two Musical Paintings* by Piet Mondrian, *Composition with Gray Lines and Victory Boogie Woogie*, figure 4.6 on page 58, © 2008 Massachusetts Institute of Technology, by permission of The MIT Press.

Chapter 7
    Baron-Cohen, Simon and Harrison, John. 1997. "Synesthesia: A Review of Psychological Theories." In *Synesthesia: Classic and Contemporary Readings*, edited by Simon Baron Cohen and John Harrison. p.121. Hoboken: Blackwell Publishing.
    Cytowic, Richard, E., M.D, *The Man Who Tasted Shapes*, p.142, short text excerpt, © 2003 Massachusetts Institute of Technology, by permission of The MIT Press.
    Duffy, Patricia Lynn. 2001. *Blue Cats and Chartreuse Kittens*, p.27, 71, New York: Henry Holt and Co.
    van Campen, Cretien, *The Hidden Sense*, p12, 57, short text excerpt, © 2008 Massachusetts Institute of Technology, by permission of The MIT Press.
    van Campen, Cretien. "Artistic and Psychological Experiments with Synesthesia." *Leonardo* 32, no. 1 (1999): 9-14. Accessed April 4, 2022. http://www.synesthesie.nl/pub/synleon99.htm.

Chapter 8
    Carla. Email message to author. 10 May, 2023.
    Cole, Rainye. "Rainye's Colorful World." Last modified: November 29, 2020. https://rainyescworld.blogspot.com/.
    Cycleoverload. "My synesthesia makes my life worth living." Reddit, 10 May, 2023. https://www.reddit.com/r/Synesthesia/comments/13c2k3a/seeking_synesthesia_participants/jjkotlk/?context= 3.

Peckover, Robin. Email message via Sean Day's synesthesia email list. 9 June, 2023

Schultze, Alice. Email message to the author via Sean Day's synesthesia email list. 9 June, 2023.

INDEX

alphabet 31, 44, 47, 55, 61-66
associative synesthesia 14, 77
auras 19
automated sensory meridian response 18
bidirectional synesthesia 6, 16
Blige, Mary J. 10
Bowerman, Jane 22
chromesthesia 14
colored hearing synesthesia 14, 17-18, 35, 78
concurrents, *See* photisms
Day, Sean 7, 21, 40, 43, 81
days of the week 7, 17, 31, 44, 47-50, 55, 66
Desana Indians 45
Diagnostic and Statistical Manual of Mental Disorders 8
flavors—color 13-15, 80
form constants 19-20
genes 21, 40
grapheme color 5-6, 9, 13, 16-18, 21, 35, 41, 43, 47, 51, 54-55, 57, 73,
grapheme personification 14, 19
homonyms 54
inheritable synesthesia 7, 11, 21, 31
intelligence, types of 43
Kandinsky, Wassily 70-71
Kluver, Heinrich 19-20
Kubin, Alfred 43
lexical-gustatory synesthesia 14, 78, 80
localizers, *See* associative synesthesia
Messiaen, Olivier 16, 22
mirror-touch synesthesia 13-14

misophonia 8, 14
Monroe, Marilyn 10
months of the year 14, 17, 44, 47, 50, 55-57, 66
music—flavors 13
non-localizers 14
numbers 9, 14, 19, 35, 38, 41, 43-44, 47-48, 55, 57-61, 64-66, 75, 79
O'Keefe, Georgia 22
pain—color 13, 41, 77
personalities—color 13
phoneme color synesthesia 13, 16, 52, 54
photisms 16, 18, 24, 31
polymodal synesthesia 15, 22
projective synesthesia 14
Scriabin, Alexander 69-71
smells—touch 13
sounds—color 6, 14, 16, 18, 35, 54, 67, 74
spatial-sequence synesthesia 14
Steen, Carol 40
Torrance Test of Creative Thinking 10
Van Gogh, Vincent 10
Watson, Michael 15, 22-23, 74
Williams, Pharrell 10
X chromosome 40

www.ingramcontent.com/pod-product-compliance
Lightning Source LLC
LaVergne TN
LVHW070940070526
838199LV00039B/724